PERFECT SUCKING

A Female Guide with Great Insight on How to Give a Man Head and Other Related Sexual Pleasures

ROSELYN DOUGLAS

TABLE OF CONTENTS

CHAPTER 1

INTRODUCTION

Sexual pleasure is that the physical and/or psychological satisfaction and pleasure derived from solitary or shared titillating experiences, as well as thoughts, dreams and automotive vehicle eroticism.

Self-determination, consent, safety, privacy, confidence and also the ability to speak and talk over sexual relations are key facultative factors for pleasure to contribute to sexual health and well being. Pleasure ought to be exercised among the context of sexual rights, significantly the rights to equality and fairness, autonomy and bodily integrity, the correct to the best getable commonplace of health and freedom of expression. The expertise of human pleasure are numerous and sexual rights make sure that pleasure may be a positive experience for all involved and not obtained by violating different people's human rights and well being.

Human sex is however folks expertise the titillating and categorical themselves as sexual beings. Human sex has several aspects. Biologically, sex refers to the fruitful mechanism similarly because the basic biological drive that exists all told species and might comprehend sexual activity and sexual contact all told its forms. There are emotional or physical sides of sex that refers to the bond that exists between people, which can be expressed through profound feelings or emotions, and which can be manifested in physical or medical issues concerning the physiological or perhaps psychological aspects of sexual behavior. Sociologically it will cowl the cultural, political, and legal aspects; and philosophically, it will span the ethical, ethical, system of rules, non secular or non secular aspects.

Recent studies on human sex have highlighted that sexual aspects are of major importance in increase personality and to social evolution of individuals:

 Human sex isn't merely obligatory by instinct or stereotypic conducts, because it happens in animals, however it's influenced each by superior mental activity and by social, cultural, instructional and normative characteristics of these places wherever the topics get older and their temperament develops. Consequently, the analysis of sexual sphere should be supported the convergence of many lines of development like fond, emotions and relations.

CHAPTER 2

WHAT IS BLOW JOB?

A blow job is once a person or lady puts their lover's member in their mouth, and yield to suck and lick it for the man's pleasure. It's conjointly referred to as sexual perversion, fellatio, or "going down on" somebody. The feminine version is named head.

CHAPTER 3

FACTORS INFLUENCING SEXUALITY IN HUMANS

Human sex is often influenced by secretion changes within the development of the vertebrate throughout maternity. Some claim its manner of expression is essentially thanks to genetic predisposition. Others say it's thanks to one's own personal experimentation in adolescence, and so the institution of preferences. A less discordant approach acknowledges that each factor might have a mutual role to play. A primary criticism of the concept that gayness is a minimum of partially genetically determined is that the proven fact that homosexual men ar less doubtless to create, which implies any genes that contribute to their sexual identity won't be passed on to offspring, suggesting the genes that contribute to their homosexual identity can die with them. But recent analysis has found that gayness might follow a "kin selection" biological process model. The essential plan of kin choice is that some people might not create, however they're going to work to facilitate the sexual practice of their relatives and therefore the survival of their relatives' offspring. By facilitating the success of their siblings' offspring, they are, indirectly, insuring the copy of their genes. In one study examining this idea, the fa'afafine of Samoa, gay men

UN agency are thought-about a definite gender class aside from either men or ladies, were found to in reality be a lot of concerned within the lives of their nieces and nephews than were heterosexual aunts and uncles. This analysis supports the kin choice model of sexual identity and helps justify why there's a genetic element to gayness even supposing homosexuals are less doubtless than heterosexuals to create.

Human sex may be understood as a part of the social lifetime of humans, ruled by implicit rules of behavior and therefore the established order. Thus, it's claimed, sex influences social norms and society successively influences the style within which sex are often expressed. Since the invention of the mass media, sex has more molded the environments within which we tend to live; it involves be distilled (often into stereotypes) then repeatedly expressed in commercial forms like print, audio and film.

Human sex is distinguished from identity. Identity could be a a lot of expansive set of roles than sexual identity. Gender will typically be molded by the social surroundings to that one is exposed as a baby, e.g. Associate in Nursing authority giving a touch boy a toy truck to play with, and a woman a doll. Human physiology and gender molding so makes sure types of sexual expression potential or maybe doubtless, however it doesn't predict that future sexual behavior are going to be considered 'gender appropriate'.

Human sexual selections are typically created exploitation current cultural norms. For example; some might like better to abstain from sex before wedding as a result of their faith forbids such actions. In some cultures it should be acceptable for a person to own several wives, whereas in others bigamy or marriage is frowned upon. Those that want to specific are dissident sex typically kind sub-cultures, inside the most culture.

CHAPTER 4

HOW GIVING A BLOW JOB LEADS TO SEXUAL PLEASURE

Oral sex will appear knotty if you think that concerning it once you are not turned on. You are imagined to place your mouth where? And you'd need someone's face in your most non-public spot why? However within the moment, once you are with somebody you are into, perversion will appear to be an additional genius invention than the light bulb. The sole annoying half is once you are having sex with a bloke and sure blow job myths get within the manner of each of you enjoying the act the maximum amount as doable.

Here are some listed blow jobs tips you need to know;

Learn to swallow even though you're not a fan:

Unlike smoothies, body fluid isn't some nutrient-rich elixir. Once you treat somebody to a mouth-induced coming, they do not get to gauge what you are doing once the very fact. Spit, swallow, move out of the manner thus it does not get in your hair, whatever. As long as you are not like, "this is often foul, you are a beast," there should not be any complaints.

Statistically, all men are obsessed with blow job, so be careful if a man doesn't want one:

There are such a big amount of reasons a man might not be up for a blow job. Rather like some ladies love receiving perversion et al. like completely different varieties of clitoris recreation, he may be into a special quite sexual practice. Or he might be saving you from encountering his wet post-workout package. Or even he needs to speak concerning his feelings rather than having sex. Point is, it does not mechanically mean he does not such as you or thinks your blow jobs are awful.

Deep throat aids an excellent blow job:

If you'll deep throat while not issue, go for it. Its associate degree awing talent that you just sadly cannot list on your resume; therefore use it after you will. However you'll conjointly provides a stellar blow job while not the top of a phallus agitating your pharyngeal reflex.

The unique blow job position:

Actually, there is a whole wide world of perversion positions out there on the far side you kneel before of him. You'll attempt sixty nine, lying next to him, your head hanging off the bed, lying down whereas he kneels on prime of you, so way more.

It is good for a man to put your head lower:

Great if it turns you on. However, if it causes you to feel weird, raise him to prevent. Blow jobs ought to be sensible for each individual, not simply the one receiving them.

A blow job isn't real sex:

For some ladies, obtaining face-to-face with an erectile organ is a lot of intimate than having PIV sex. And though you are not one in all them, you'll be able to positively still get sexually transmitted infections from giving a blow job as a result of you are exchanging bodily fluids and you'll be able to conjointly get STIs like herpes and HPV from skin-to-skin contact).

Your teeth might make the penis to fall off:

The world will not finish as a result of you expertise a bit teeth penis contact. As long as you are not scraping them up and down his shaft throughout, it's in all probability not a problem. Looking on the guy, he would possibly even like it! However undoubtedly rise before doing it by choice.

You have to perform a blow job to it completion:

You could. Otherwise you might trade off, thus he goes down on you for a touch, and then you continue giving him a blow job once. Otherwise you might stop before he comes and pair tills his orgasms. Otherwise you might split intercourse with some bouts of sexual perversion. The top goal does not continually need to be consummation.

Your mouth should provide enough spit to make the act enjoyable:

Cotton mouth happens. Luckily, tasteful make full exists! Simply make certain to use a sort that is compatible with condoms if they seem to be a part of your sex routine, and conjointly confirm it's safe for intercourse if you propose on doing that once.

You need blow-job sorcery for uncircumcised penises.

An uncircumcised erectile organ remains cased in its foreskin, which covers the top. A circumcised erectile organ now not incorporates a foreskin, therefore the head is exposed. That is the solely difference they're each still penises, and guys still adore it after you bit them.

If you seize on the way, you need to start afresh:

If he is right the brink of coming and you decision a trip, yes, you'll likely ought to place in some further work to induce him back to the purpose of no come back. However if you are feeling like your jaw's seizing up, provides it a rest. You'll be able to use your hands to stay the nice feelings going.

You just need to love giving blow job to stay sexy:

You know that World Health Organizational plan of however nothing's hotter than a girl who loves giving blow jobs such a lot; she will be able too much coming from them? False Enthusiasm is usually enticing; however you ought not to worship at the blow job altar to

be enticing yourself.

CHAPTER 5

WHAT YOU SHOULD KNOW REGARDING THE INTIMACY OF ORAL SEX TO SEX

In here, I will be explaining more about the satisfactory level regarding oral sex to merely sex which most folks do engage in and most likely will lead to some issues in relationship or marital homes:

Oral sex is foreplay while sex is just an instant gratification:

If you are drunk at a bar and you are taking somebody home, you are not planning to take the time to travel down on this randomly. You are going to let him stick his dick within you and flail around wildly before collapsing on your body.

That's all a one-night stand very is, anyway: swing the P within the V. desirous to get yours and obtain out.

Oral sex is sex. It takes exactitude and dedication. Once was the last time you gave associate adequate, drunk blowjob? Certain, you may have popped his d*ck in your mouth for some seconds throughout your intoxicated makes an attempt to be attractive; however that is in all probability it.

In oral sex, your focal point is the satisfactory level of your partner and not yourself:

Sexual intercourse is generally inconsiderate. Sure, you wish the opposite person to induce off; however your own climax is your initial priority.

But giving head is, at the core, a unselfish act. Also, there isn't any position additional vulnerable than being on your knees.

If you are giving a fellation, you are serving this different person with no guarantee that you're going to receive identical satisfaction. You are abandoning your pleasure and maybe suffering some discomfort -- for the sake of constructing somebody else happy. You are valuing another person's pleasure higher than your own.

You're showing him you genuinely care that he feels smart. You do not care solely regarding yourself.

And albeit you are giving head to induce head, you've got to trust that the opposite person goes to come back the favor, which cannot continuously happen.

You're clearly banking plenty on this person, which is intimate in and of it.

Being on your knees is actually the best position:

With sex, you are equals. You each management the extent of intimacy during this encounter, and you are each obtaining one thing out of it.

But giving head mechanically puts another person au fait. You are within the submissive position.

You have to trust a man enough to feel snug matures your knees and golf stroke his erectile organ in your mouth. You've got to trust him to not treat you wish garbage throughout or when the act.

By agreeing to relinquish him head, you are demonstrating that you simply have religion in your relationship and believe he is a decent person.

Oral sex requires complete focus while sex could be thoughtless:

Sex is impersonal, anonymous and transitory.

But perversion needs dedication and focus. It is a job that takes talent. And if you are giving head, you are specializing in sharing your skills for your partner's profit.

Oral sex is not one thing that may be taken gently. One wrong move with perversion, and somebody may get hurt (think: teeth), as a result of it is a sex that needs your attention and warm-heartedness.

When you're putting so much effort in the work, you obviously like the person:

If I am supplying you with a fellation, you'll be able to bet your blue balls that I actually have a factor for you. i do not feel the requirement to place in any further effort for a gallant i do not require to put in so much effort towards someone I do not care about. If I would like to travel down on you, it's as a result of i prefer you.

If somebody is willing to place sexual arousal on the backburner for the delight of a partner, that is an indication of warm-heartedness. If you are deep-throating a man, you are into him. Why else wrestle such

a task?

THE END

www.ingramcontent.com/pod-product-compliance
Lightning Source LLC
Chambersburg PA
CBHW050751250726
48662CB00005B/2167